The Advantage
of
Powerful Lungs

Author and Publisher
Earle E. Liederman
305 Broadway · New York

THE ADVANTAGE OF POWERFUL LUNGS

(ORIGINAL VERSION, RESTORED)

By

EARLE LIEDERMAN

Original Publisher: Earle Liederman, 305 Broadway, New York, 1927

PUBLISHED BY O'Faolain Patriot LLC, Copyright 2011

info@PhysicalCultureBooks.com

ISBN-13: 978-1467977807

ISBN-10: 1467977802

Published in the United States of America

To Order More Copies Visit: Physical Culture Books.com

THE ADVANTAGE OF POWERFUL LUNGS

ABILITY brought on by practice, endurance, fatigue, and recuperative powers all are closely linked together. No one can make good, whether he be a runner, boxer or athlete in any other sport, unless his organs as well as his muscles work in harmony, and unless the muscles possess the ability to recuperate between exercises. A beginner's muscles will sadly lack these qualities, and largely because of the lack of acquired coordination through overcoming the antagonistic muscles. Naturally, in such a condition fatigue sets in.

Often deer chased by huntsmen have been known to drop dead from exhaustion; but during exercise a human muscle never reaches the condition of absolute fatigue or complete powerlessness. This is prevented by the painful sensation experienced before the muscle becomes absolutely incapable of action. The rest that is enforced by the thoroughly aching muscle checks the further development of fatigue. Even should the enthusiast desire to continue the movement after the muscle is aching, the pain and suffering soon would become so intense as to eliminate all forced action by will power.

I once read what was an excellent illustration proving that muscles really never become absolutely exhausted. It also was stated that all the will power a man may possess cannot exhaust the last remaining power still left in a muscle after it reaches the severely aching point. As nearly as I can recall it, it read something like this: One of the most tiring attitudes to assume is that which consists of holding the arms outstretched horizontally. The deltoid or shoulder muscle does most of the work. There are very few who are vigorous enough to hold the arms in this manner for more than five or six minutes. At the end of this time the deltoids cannot act any longer and the arms drop. But the muscles are not exhausted; the fibres still possess a great contractive force. This can be proven by the fact that certain stimulants, such as electricity, can bring into play this motive force over which the will no longer has any action. If by waiting until the sensation of fatigue becomes unbearable to a man who is holding out his arms, and if at the moment when he declares he has used up all his power and is about to let his arms fall, you apply a strong electric current to the shoulder muscles the fatigue and feebleness seem to vanish and the arms remain outstretched, showing that the muscles have not lost all their contractile power.

It is undesirable to work a muscle to such a degree that an abnormal stimulant is required to bring forth further contractions. It is wise to discontinue the movement and to relax when, or even before, the aching point begins to develop. After a time it will be found that you will not have as many aches as you used to have, and these, of course, are eradicated by practice and experience in the various movements and by the development of better tone— better endurance—in the muscles themselves. The more experience you have in a certain movement the more endurance you will acquire. Do you think for one instant that a mountain climber could continue until he reaches the summit if it were his first attempt? Naturally, the first time he climbed anything he would experience fatigue; but by constant practice he finally is able to avoid this fatigue by having his muscles in condition and working in coordination.

One year while in Seward, Alaska, I stood gazing at quite a high mountain on whose round top there had been placed a flag. I inquired of a passerby for what purpose the flag had been put there. He told me the mountain was known as Marathon Mountain, and that each year there was an annual race up to this flag pole and back, the winner being presented with a prize. I almost opened my mouth in astonishment, for it was hard to realize how a human being could run up the side of such a heavy grade and for so long a distance, for this mountain must have been fully four thousand feet in height. If any one of you have tried to run uphill you will appreciate the wonderful endurance it takes to run the short distance of even one hundred yards. I feel quite certain that those who participate in this annual Marathon Mountain run would not think of making the attempt without first rehearsing at least a good distance up the slope, and regularly, for several or many days before the race.

Anyone who wishes to experiment in uphill running should try running two or three steps at a time up the stairway of a tall office building. I am sure he would find himself extremely tired long before reaching the top, and I would not recommend such exertion to anyone who has not conditioned his legs, heart and lungs beforehand, by first practicing one flight, two flights a day later, and progressively to the top in this manner. It would be foolhardy for anyone to attempt it otherwise; for not only would fatigue set in, but the heart action would be greatly disturbed, possibly the heart damaged, and most likely serious consequences would follow.

The power to resist fatigue is essential in acquiring endurance, and, in fact, may be said to constitute endurance. If you have refrained from exercise for some time and your body suffers for the want of it, fatigue well may be dreaded; whereas, if you exercise daily and keep your body in good condition you will have no cause to dread fatigue. But by having too long periods of repose, such as omitting your exercising drills for days at a time, it will make you more susceptible to muscular fatigue and muscle lameness than if you daily performed physical activities for but a few minutes. Therefore, it is essential, as I have so many times stated, always to be in good condition.

The only way to gain the power to resist fatigue is to increase power and endurance of muscles, heart and lungs. You must continue each day whatever exertions you are performing, until the muscles begin to feel tired. After a while what exertions once brought on fatigue and demanded relaxation no longer will do so. In time you can continue with the activity without thought of fatigue, and for what, to the inactive person, will be an almost unbelievable length of time.

A well-trained man resists fatigue easily, not because he ignores the painful sensations which usually or frequently accompany work, but because these sensations are not produced in him, or at most are produced in very slight and easily variable degree. Exercise induces nutrition in all the tissues of the body. This makes them more resistant and firmer, and, in a sense, arms them against shocks and friction and protects them against the accidents of work. On the contrary, prolonged repose makes the tissues softer and more susceptible to the shocks and accidents.

Fatigue in all its forms is felt especially after too much rest has been taken. If anyone has had the experience of traveling across the country, from coast to coast, he will realize more than ever the value of daily exercise. I have taken this trip numerous times and, while I always keep myself in excellent condition, a three- or four-day ride on the trains, with its dusty or super-heated atmosphere and lack of activity, makes me feel, upon arriving at my destination, that my energies have been lowered appreciably.

Once, after I had been in heavy active training for several months, I went from New York to Seattle, Wash. After leaving my baggage at my hotel, I took a walk up and down the hills of various streets. Anyone who has been to Seattle will know what steep grades there are along some of the side streets which cross the main thoroughfares. I found in time that upon reaching the tops of these little hilly streets I was beginning to puff, when ordinarily I would not have been so affected by such exercise. This breathless condition was brought on by my four-day train ride, during which I had practically no physical activity whatever. This indicates the importance of allowing no day to elapse without doing exercise in some form or another.

My belief is that in these modern times the automobile takes a great many years from people's lives. How many business men are there who upon leaving their homes walk to the elevator of their apartment or hotel, which carries them down to the street and there awaits their car, which brings them direct to the office where they again enter an elevator, which brings them practically to,their desk? After a day of inactivity they ride home; and they repeat this same routine day after day. It is no wonder they become fat and flabby, with absolutely no endurance. They would suffer from lameness and stiffness if they walked the length of two or three blocks. Finally they wonder what their troubles may be. Perhaps, upon advice from their physician, they decide upon an hour's walk. They probably are in bed with fever the next morning. But take the postman, who walks and stands continuously all day long. He goes to bed without feeling any ill effects from the exertion, and awakes in the morning feeling fully fit for his duties.

The fatigue which follows an exercise of speed is unlike that experienced after an exercise of strength. In performing strength work the muscular contraction is well in evidence and is slow and prolonged, and the fatigue is especially felt in the muscle. The limbs become weary and congested. The blood flows to them and swells them, which is usually the most encouraging thing a physical culture enthusiast can experience. When I first began exercising, I performed my work before a mirror, and I was just as enthusiastic about my measurements and increasing the size of my muscles as my pupils are today. I actually measured my muscles every day to see whether or not they were increasing in size. How encouraged I felt when, upon finishing a certain movement and measuring the muscle which performed the movement, I found that it had increased about one-quarter of an inch in size; and how disappointed I was when later in the day I found I had lost the one-quarter of an inch, as the blood had left the muscle, naturally decreasing the size of the muscle. But the constant swelling up or bringing of blood to the part used by the activity of the exercise positively will increase its size permanently, if not overdone to the point of exhaustion of cells, energy and building material.

The expression "nervous fatigue" gives a good idea of the kind of disturbance which easily is recognized by those who have ever prolonged an exercise of speed. There is less desire for sleep, and the appetite also lessens. These effects are produced by the great expenditure of nervous energy, which an exercise of speed makes necessary and which makes the repair of the exercised structures more difficult. Speed work, also, will take off weight, which can be laid to the expenditure of nervous energy in performing the speed work, just as any nervous strain upon the body is bound to reduce the weight.

While fatigue may be muscular or nervous, it also can be mental and take the form of depression. This depression can be created by overwork and by using the will power to force the muscles beyond their natural tiring point. It is interesting to note what stimulating effect the mind has upon the muscles, especially when they are fatigued. Those who have engaged in actual warfare know what aching and swollen feet mean upon returning from the trenches, exhausted and depressed because of the tremendous amount of nerve force and muscular action used in advancing and in retiring in combat. It is a common sight to see comrades dropping exhausted, one by one, on their return march. But let someone shout, "the enemy is coming," and everyone will be on his feet, forgetful of fatigue and depression.

It will be seen, therefore, that besides our will power forcing our muscles onward, that additional stimulus can be created by fear and excitement. Of course, greater reaction is bound to follow when such added stimulus compels further muscular action. But whether it be fear of bodily injury or fear of losing out, such mental stimulus will prove very interesting in the study of endurance work. It is not wise to force the muscles by the will to such a degree as is possible by some emotion unless a life or a great accomplishment depends upon it; and except in some crisis or urgent need it is well to discontinue movement when the feeling of tiredness enters the muscles involved. Muscles should be in such condition that fatigue would not manifest itself, through training and possessing the ability to recuperate between movements. And again let me repeat there probably will be lack of recuperative power if relaxation between movements is not secured, or if coordination is defective and muscle antagonism plays the chief role during the movements.

The sensation of fatigue prevents one from having an exact idea of the energy which the muscular fibres still possess; and it compels rest long before all the force of the muscles has been spent, just as hunger warns us that we need food long before the body becomes weakened from lack of nourishment. The sensation of fatigue should put us on guard. As I have said, it would be dangerous to continue working until the muscles become completely exhausted and incapable of contracting, and we should look upon early signs of fatigue as nature's warning to discontinue all movement.

The student will find that a greater number of movements can be made if the mind centers on other things. If you think about what you are doing the concentration on the movement naturally will tire your muscles quicker than if your mind wanders. Mental concentration while exercising, therefore, can be seen to be better for muscle building than for endurance work. As an organ, the heart is an example of this. It beats throughout our lives. Its movements are involuntary, just as are the movements of the lungs. Neither the heart nor the lungs ever determines* the sensation of fatigue in individual muscles or groups of muscles.

The muscles ordinarily under the control of the will have the same immunity to fatigue if their contraction is made more or less involuntary. This easily can be observed in patients suffering from St. Vitus' Dance or those suffering from palsy. In either case movement after movement is performed against the will, from morning till night, and yet muscular fatigue does not develop in appreciable degree. If an athlete were to continue such a series of movements, impelling himself to do so by force of will, complete exhaustion would set in before many hours would pass.

The student will find for himself that an exercise which is accompanied by concentration, that is with the thought on every movement he is doing, will prove more fatiguing than a movement which is performed independently of the will. Again may be mentioned the beginner with his lack of coordination and muscle sense and who is wholly dependent upon his enthusiasm and desire to achieve in a difficult sport or pastime. The tension he puts forth with each effort can be likened to the most strenuous muscle-building for the experienced athlete.

It is a known fact that good lungs are essential for endurance. The one who has the best "wind" usually wins the long distance or long drawn out event. As you know, the essential condition of breathing is the presence in the lungs of air and blood. The oxygen in the air purifies the blood that is pumped by the heart through the blood vessels. However, this is physiology, which can be found in any book on that subject.

Have you ever found yourself within sight of the railroad station and afraid of missing your train? There probably was a quarter of a mile still to go and your watch showed that there was less than two minutes till train departure. You rushed to make it. For months you had been accustomed to use the same gait, perhaps, in walking to the station. However, in this instance you have had to pluck up courage and run, or else wait for the next train. Perhaps you were in fairly good condition—your legs quite strong. However, after a few seconds a peculiar distress came on. Your breathing became difficult and your chest felt heavy. Mayhap you caught the train, but what happened after you entered the car? As the train started you sank almost exhausted upon the cushions. In spite of the fact that your exertion had ended, your distress continued. For some minutes you were out of breath — winded. You may have been surprised when you considered that though your legs were strong yet your lungs or heart appeared weak. Your legs did the real work, why didn't they feel the fatigue first? But every time you work your legs you also give your lungs and heart an added amount of work; and in endurance tests it is these organs that first feel the strain, in those who are unprepared by graduated systematic and regular exercise.

I am a firm advocate of deep breathing and giving the lungs plenty of work. The more often you take deep inhalations through the day the larger your rib-box will become and the greater will be your lung capacity; but deep breathing alone, while sitting, walking or standing, will have no direct increasing effect whatever upon endurance. If you desire to possess wind—that staying power that will enable you to reach your goal in endurance activities—you must go through the actual practice in the sport in which you expect to excel. Deep breathing taken at various intervals throughout the day will, of course, help considerably in increasing capacity and strength of the lungs but it will not bring you endurance.

I doubt whether anyone has a better lung capacity than most opera singers. They have mastered the art of breath control and are able to breathe so systematically yet unconsciously that it in no way interferes with their singing; in fact, their ability to breathe properly makes possible their superior singing. They are able to hold their notes for an astonishing length of time. Yet they would make a poor showing in any form of endurance work if they have never practiced that particular activity.

While attending normal school, studying to become a teacher when I first became interested in this work, I frequently played handball and squash with one of the Metropolitan Opera House bassos. Now, handball is a game that will "wind" one very quickly unless he becomes proficient in this pastime. By becoming proficient I mean experienced in the practice. This basso (whose name is immaterial here) appeared to be in excellent condition. His shoulders were broad, his body erect, and he possessed great depth to his chest. His arms and legs, also, had pleasing curves, which indicated that he had kept himself in excellent condition by some form or other of exercise. But he had done no running, and it was evident to me, after playing one game of handball with him and watching him pant for breath, that all the exercising he had done consisted of movements performed while standing stationary. He probably had squatted up and down for his thighs, rose up and down on his toes for the muscles below the knee and swung his arms to and fro, possibly with Indian clubs or dumb-bells, to develop his upper body. He was sadly in need of endurance work. Perhaps such work did not appeal to him, and as musicians and singers seem to live in a world of their own, perhaps he felt that endurance would not better in the least his singing ability.

Breathlessness is a general effect—a result of the total quantity of work performed by the muscles used in an exercise. On the other hand, muscular fatigue is but a local effect. It is localized and in direct proportion to the share in the work taken by each muscle used in the exercise. When the work is too light to produce breathlessness, it can produce fatigue if your effort is performed by a small group of muscles or by groups of very weak muscles. But if your exercises involve a great number of muscles or are performed by large muscle groups, the effort you put forth will be too great to produce local muscular fatigue and, therefore, you will find yourself breathless—winded.

Breathlessness is caused partly by the over-driving of the heart, and by the congestion of the lungs which this immediately produces. When you perform an exercise calling for a maximum or prolonged effort, you will find that breathlessness comes on with astonishing rapidity.

If you run upstairs you will find breathlessness occurring much sooner than when you run on the level ground. In certain muscular actions fatigue takes the form of breathlessness, and the respiratory distress forces you to stop exercising long before the muscles themselves are fatigued. You can swing your arms, for example, or exercise with light dumb-bells, following the old-fashioned dumb-bell drill, and continue until your arms are aching, and yet you will not be winded. This explains why a well-developed man, whose shoulders are broad, whose deltoids are rounded, and whose pectorals and upper arms have beautiful contour, may not necessarily be any good when it comes to endurance. He may have developed his upper muscular body without developing his lungs. But, if this same muscular individual has firm, well-rounded thighs and well formed muscular hips, you can rest assured that his lungs are in Al condition; for it is practically impossible for one to perform vigorous leg movements without bringing into play all the "wind" or lung power and capacity that he possesses.

Try the simple experiment of holding your arm out sideways. You will find that after about four or five minutes you will be compelled to lower it, and yet your breathing will be normal. Try the same exercise, holding in your hand a pair of three-pound or five-pound dumb-bells; still, even after your det- toids are thoroughly aching, you will find your breathing about the same as before you began the test. You may be obliged to stop these light upper- body exercises, not because you are out of breath but because your muscular or nerve force has been expended.

An authority on exercise once heard a horse trainer say, "A horse trots with his legs and gallops with his lungs." This expresses well the importance of pace in the production of breathlessness. Why should a horse be more out of breath after a gallop than after a trot? The first thought would be to attribute the more prompt breathlessness to the greater swiftness, but we must not become confused between pace and speed. You can slow down the gallop of a horse until it falls behind another horse which may be trotting. There are some horses, as you know, so awkward that their gallop is as slow as a fast walk. However, no matter how slow a gallop may be the horse will become out of breath quicker than he would from an equally rapid trot. This is because more muscles are used at the same instant, the movements are more rapid even if the pace is not, and the entire weight is lifted from the ground at once, very frequently.

. Therefore, one does not become breathless under the same conditions as produce local muscular fatigue, such as exercising the muscles singly, tiring the biceps alone as by curling, or the deltoids alone as by raising the arms sideways. It is true that it is impossible to exercise the arms, for example, without working the shoulders, the back and the chest to a considerable extent. Even though you concentrate wholly upon arm work, the muscles of your back and shoulders will be exercised to some extent by the arm movement. In spite of this, you will find that your muscles will tire long before you become winded. If you want to see the difference between twenty-five movements performed by the muscles of the upper body and twenty-five movements performed by the muscles below the waist, just do any exercise you may choose for the muscles above the waist for twenty-five counts and then jump as high as you can twenty-five times without stopping, and note the difference in your breathing after these two exercises.

The peculiarity in the breathlessness caused by heavy leg exercises is not that it is hard to inhale, but that it is hard to exhale all the air from the lungs. No better instance of this can be had than in swimming. It is a very easy matter when swimming the crawl stroke to inhale as much air in one gulp as is needed; but you will find when you turn your head sideways for your next inhalation that, unless you are an expert in the art of breathing, all the air will not have been exhaled from your lungs and you cannot inhale much. This breathing difficulty is one reason why very few of us care to become long distance swimmers. Breathing while swimming is an art which must be mastered, and there is not one swimmer in a hundred who has fully mastered it. These are the ones who swim a mile or two with small effort and at the end find themselves breathing just as normally as when they started.

Upon investigating the condition common to all muscular activities which are said to be capable of rapidly producing respiratory troubles, you will find that all movements that require a great expenditure of force produce breathlessness. Of course, breathlessness can be produced by holding the breath, and anyone who has endeavored to swim under water for any distance realizes when he has to come up for air that he needs it badly, also that he is somewhat winded. This is a voluntarily created breathlessness. I would not advise anyone to see how long he can hold his breath, for such a willful respiratory disturbance interferes with the heart action, circulation, and general health.

The condition of the extensor muscles of the thigh, and the other muscles of the legs as well, have a good deal to do with wind. For instance, if you trot at a certain rhythmic pace, let us say for a distance of a quarter of a mile, you will not be as winded as you would be if, while keeping the same rhythmic pace, you sprang higher into the air or put more effort into each leg movement. In other words, the more effort placed upon the leg muscles, the quicker you become winded, even though you do not change the timing or the pace. This is because the greater effort greatly increases heart action and circulation and makes a greater demand upon the lungs for oxygen to take care of the larger quantity of blood passing through them at a more rapid rate. More nervous energy is used, and, too, the interest usually is more deeply aroused when one is undergoing more rapid exercise. These all affect the wind.

Another illustration is deep knee-bending exercise. You can squat and raise for, perhaps, one hundred or more repetitions before you feel slightly out of breath. (I am taking it for granted, of course, that you are in good condition.) Just try and do the same exercise but, instead of simply raising the body by the strength of your thighs, push off the ground vigorously and jump into the air. You will find that your respiratory organs will feel the effects of these latter efforts much sooner than the former.

To determine for yourself which of certain movements produce local fatigue and which movements produce breathlessness, sit on a chair and rotate your feet around in circles until the muscles of your shin become paralyzed from fatigue. This is an example of local fatigue. Next have someone sit on your shoulders or else have a bar-bell resting on your shoulders, and perform the squatting exercise; that is, bend your knees until you almost sit on your heels, and then rise again until your legs are straight. You will find after a comparatively few number of repetitions that you will be breathless, because you have used larger muscles strenuously in groups. You have worked the thighs, the calves, the back, and even the abdominal muscles in the performance of these movements. If you desire to develop endurance, it is much better to perform exercises that produce breathlessness than it is to carry out movements that simply produce local fatigue.

If you exercise the muscles singly, that is one at a time, until each one is thoroughly tired, you may develop them; but they will lack coordination and the muscle sense that will be required in performing endurance work. On the other hand, if you exercise the muscles in groups, you naturally induce breathlessness much sooner, but at least you are working them in harmony and coordination, and at the same time you are increasing your lung power, which will be needed in all endurance pastimes.

When an exercise causes breathlessness it is not wholly due to the contraction or usage of certain muscles or the disturbance of certain organs during the exercise. It is due largely to the excessive expenditure of force which the exercise necessitates. Breathlessness occurs whenever muscular work produces in a given time more carbonic acid in the blood than the lungs can eliminate in the same time. The quantity of work necessary to produce breathlessness, then, will not be the same in all persons, for all cannot eliminate from the lungs the same quantity of carbonic acid in the same length of time. Therefore, in order to avoid becoming breathless during an exercise you must regulate the work of the muscles by the eliminating power of the lungs, in such a manner that the quantity of carbonic acid produced in a given time shall not be greater than that which the respiratory organs can dispose of during the same time.

Naturally, a man or an animal will adopt a pace in running from which he cannot materially depart without producing breathlessness. If a fairly violent exercise is performed continuously for an appreciable length of time, breathlessness always is produced in the end, even though the individual does not exceed his natural pace. If, for example, you can run at a moderate pace for five minutes without losing your breath, you will find breathlessness occurring in a quarter of an hour, even though you do not change your pace in the least. That is because, even though the work you are doing remains the same, the demand upon the lung power will become greater by the continuance of the movement, and the circulation of the blood through the lungs becomes increased.

A beginner in taking a cold shower usually makes plenty of noise. The shock of the water suddenly striking his body compels him to gasp for breath, and his respiratory organs are forced to undergo considerable activity. After a while, however, he becomes used to it and, of course, in time his body will require a greater shock to produce the same respiratory activity as occurred when the water struck his body early in this experience.

Every violent physical sensation, wherever situated, will react upon the lungs, just as any powerful emotion also will makes its influence felt. Every time the rhythm of breathing is much disturbed, breathlessness is produced, even when you may be in the condition of muscular repose. The observing student will find that if his mind is disturbed by worry or the like while going through his exercising, breathlessness will come quicker than if his mind were at ease.

It readily can be seen that another essential point toward endurance is composure of mind. Worry will bring on fatigue quicker than anything else. If, while performing movements, you are worrying about the form in which you are doing them or are thinking too much about the muscles involved, you positively will tire much more rapidly than you would if you mentally relax, the only thing on your mind being your destination or goal.

An excellent illustration showing how breathlessness will hinder your physical activity can be gotten from anyone's own life. How many times have you become provoked at someone? Unconsciously your fist may have clenched and you had a "chip on your shoulder," so to speak, ready to begin hostilities at any moment. You may not have observed it, but if you will recall the way you felt, you will recall that there was great interference with your breathing. The mental disturbance acting upon the general nervous system in that case produced respiratory disturbances.

Many people are greatly affected by shock, a sudden shock causing such a state of breathlessness as to make a person more or less gasp for air. There is a striking resemblance between the respiratory disturbance due to a violent moral impression and that which results from a powerful physical sensation. The man running, the man under a cold shower for the first time, and the man overpowered by fear, experience a kind of shock in the region of the nerve centers which preside over the respiratory movements. Therefore, in order to acquire endurance you must have the respiratory system working in perfect order, and not easily disturbed by various influences. The mind should be free from emotional disturbances, and there should be harmony of thought.

The one chief difficulty experienced by endurance athletes is breathing; and especially, strange as it may seem, the exhalation of the air. If during a run you keep the same rhythmic pace, you will find that more steps will be taken while inhaling than while exhaling. This is the case if you are breathing naturally. But after you stop running you will find just the reverse—the exhalations will be longer than the inhalations.

Those of you with experience in weight lifting will know this only too well. I have attended many contests in weight lifting and in some have acted as a judge, and, therefore, have had ample opportunity to observe the various physiological results from this pastime. I remember that while acting as a judge in one contest a strong man who possessed a very powerful build performed the lift of "two hands anyhow." This lift consisted of raising an enormous bar-bell to arms' length overhead with as many stops between the floor and straight arms overhead as the lifter desired to make. He first brought the weight to the height of his knees, and rested the bar thereon by slightly bending his legs. Next, with a tremendous heave, he brought the bell to the upper part of his thighs and held it there, while assuming a slightly squatting position. With another mighty heave he brought the bell to his belt line, there resting it on the belt and securing it in the fatty folds of his abdomen. The next tremendous effort brought the bell to the height of his shoulders and there it was locked by the strength of his arms and balanced on his upper chest. During each one of these series of lifts he took a deep inhalation and had to hold his breath during each ascent. Finally, with a mighty upward jerk he pushed the bell upwards about a foot or so, quickly bending his knees and ducking under the weight and then standing erect while holding the weight at full arms' length overhead. After balancing it there for a moment he let the bell drop heavily to the floor, and while doing so the air came out of his lungs with a roar that could be likened to the gushing of an oil well. His respiratory system was affected for a short time afterwards and his breathing was done under difficulty.

Here is an example of effort in practically only one feat of strength performed, yet the nervous concentration, plus the physical exertion, created breathlessness, while the entire performance was of not over one minute's duration. Every exercise which demands a series of efforts at short intervals for even a short period of time very quickly produces maximum effort of the heart and possibly fatigue of that organ, and affects the respiratory organs.